Herbal Remedies Guide: Uses of 100 Herbs for Common Ailments

Step-By-Step Guide for Using Herbal Remedies

Angela Curtis

I want to dedicate this to my family. Thanks for all the support you gave me while I put together this book. You guys are awesome.

Copyright © 2014 by Speedy Publishing LLC

All rights reserved. No part of this publication may be reproduced, distributed or transmitted in any form or by any means, including photocopying, recording, or other electronic or mechanical methods, without the prior written permission of the publisher, except in the case of brief quotations embodied in critical reviews and certain other noncommercial uses permitted by copyright law. For permission requests, write to the publisher, addressed "Attention: Permissions Coordinator," at the address below.

Speedy Publishing LLC (c) 2014
40 E. Main St., #1156
Newark, DE 19711
www.speedypublishing.co

Ordering Information:
Quantity sales; Special discounts are available on quantity purchases by corporations, associations, and others. For details, contact the "Special Sales Department" at the address above.

-- 1st edition

Manufactured in the United States of America

Table of Contents

Publisher's Notes i

Chapter 1: Understanding What Herbal Remedies Are 1

Chapter 2: Herbal Remedies For Common Illnesses 6

Chapter 3: Herbal Remedies For Allergies 13

Chapter 4: Dealing With Digestive Problems 16

Chapter 5: General Problems 21

Chapter 6: Why I Love Flaxseed Oil 25

Meet the Author 27

Publisher's Notes

Disclaimer

This publication is intended to provide helpful and informative material. It is not intended to diagnose, treat, cure, or prevent any health problem or condition, nor is intended to replace the advice of a physician. No action should be taken solely on the contents of this book. Always consult your physician or qualified health-care professional on any matters regarding your health and before adopting any suggestions in this book or drawing inferences from it.

The author and publisher specifically disclaim all responsibility for any liability, loss or risk, personal or otherwise, which is incurred as a consequence, directly or indirectly, from the use or application of any contents of this book.

Any and all product names referenced within this book are the trademarks of their respective owners. None of these owners have sponsored, authorized, endorsed, or approved this book.

Always read all information provided by the manufacturers' product labels before using their products. The author and publisher are not responsible for claims made by manufacturers.

Print Edition 2014

Chapter 1: Understanding What Herbal Remedies Are

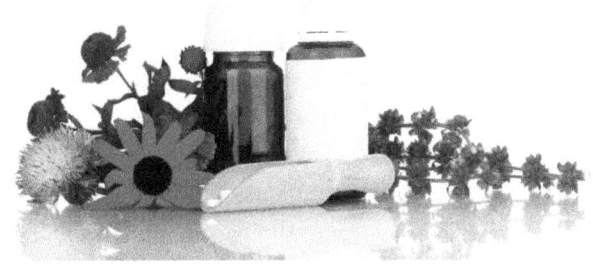

People have made use of plant extracts for centuries as a form of treating illnesses. Just a mere three thousand five hundred years ago the Egyptians were making use of herbal remedies. There is also evidence to show that other ancient nations such as the Indians, Chinese, Persians and tribes in the Americas also made use of medicinal herbs.

No one can really confirm who made use of plants for medicinal purposes first. If you are observant you will see that even animals eat certain plants when they are ill so this process could have been in existence before human history.

The stories of herbal folklore have gone through its own evolution as remedies have been passed down through families. Things went viral (so to speak) with the invention of the printing press and the ability to print and distribute various herbal recipes became possible.

By the time we got to the seventeenth century the first book, Complete Herbal (1653), was published by Nicholas Culpeper. As time went on it became increasingly evident that herbal remedies had its place in healthcare; it is the preferred method of treatment for many. Even doctors are going back to basics where treatment of particular illnesses is concerned.

Herbal Medicine - How Does It Work?

Instead of basing their method of treatment on the individual symptoms, herbalists concentrate on the underlying cause of the illness. The premise is that the use of herbal tonics and tinctures will help the body to heal itself and regain its "life force".

This leads us to the term herbal synergy. This is the term on which herbal medicine is based. This medicine tends to be a combination of extracts from petals, leaves and the roots of plants. In contrast, a typical chemical based treatment will contain one active ingredient. Herbal synergy is the combination of numerous natural extracts to treat the underlying cause of an illness.

Many of the drugs sold in pharmacies today were actually based on extracts. A prime example is the drug ephedrine which was first found in the herb Ephedra. As the tablet only contains one compound it has the side effect of raising the users' blood pressure. The herbalist will point out that there is also a compound in the plant that helps counteract that side effect, and as such, the herbal remedy is better as it not only treats the chest issues but has the components to keep the users blood pressure from being elevated.

The Treatment Process - What Happens?

When an individual has a consult with an herbalist they will go through the problem that brought them there in first place: medical history, current dietary and lifestyle habits and from that create a profile. This will typically take about an hour.

After the consultation is complete the herbalist will then put medical history and information together and create a mixture that will help the patient with their symptoms. Enough will be made to last until the next appointment. If that is not the case then the patient will be advised where they can get more. Of course there is no herbal remedy that tastes great as they tend to contain a lot of compounds that are bitter to the taste.

The point to note here is that conventional methods are not totally ignored and might recommend a consult with a traditional doctor depending on the situation.

With that said, what exactly can herbal medicine help with?

- Asthma
- Arthritis
- Cold sores
- Certain types of depression
- Problems with digestion
- Eczema
- Allergies and hay fever
- Problems with menopause and menstruation

Are There Any Studies To Quantify This?

Over the years there have been quite a number of trials that have shown how effective herbal remedies really are. A prime example would be the research presented in the Lancet on St. John's Wort. It proved that this was just as effective in treating depression as a chemically based anti-depressant.

There are other remedies like ginger and garlic that have been said to help with a range of problems like digestive issues, high cholesterol and heart disease. The challenge that many of these claims have is that a lot of studies remain inconclusive.

How Does It Relate To Conventional Medicine?

It may be a bit odd to say this but a lot of the traditional pharmaceuticals being sold today sprung from discoveries in herbal medicine. For example, Willow bark led to the creation of aspirin. A drug for heart patients known as Digoxin is derived from poisonous herbs quinine and foxglove, and morphine is an extract from the opium poppy.

In general, doctors opt to go with the manufactured pharmaceuticals as there still is a lot that is not known about the long term effects of herbal remedy use. A lot of the remedies can actually be quite toxic to the body if not taken correctly. One may also become confused when having to make selections from a number of brands on display in a health food store. Some brands may have more concentrated levels of herbs than others so care needs to be taken.

Other Considerations and Cautions

Speak To a Doctor First

It does not matter how safe herbal remedies are it is best to consult with a doctor before starting any remedy as after all they are still classified as medicine. Also bear in mind that these remedies are not one shot cures to a particular problem but just serve as another way to alleviate the symptoms of your condition.

Dosage

When you consult with your doctor they can advise of the recommended dosage for particular herbal remedies especially if it is being taken in combination with other medications. This is essential to prevent any accidents. One must also be very careful when it comes to children.

Research

It is essential you learn everything you can about the product you are about to take. An informed decision is always the best one. As long as you are aware of what you are doing then you will take the herbal remedy as it should be taken. Always read the labels and make note of the ingredients to ensure that you are not allergic to any of them.

Be Cautious Of New Remedies

When you get a new remedy never take the full dosage - take half the dose to see how you react to it. If after three days or so there are no adverse effects then you can begin to take the full dosage. If there are any adverse like nausea or diarrhea stop taking it immediately.

Chapter 2: Herbal Remedies For Common Illnesses

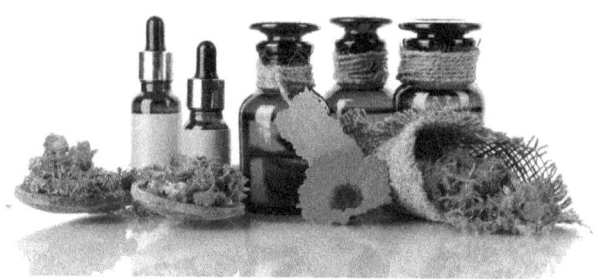

Arthritis

There are quite a number of herbal remedies used in the treatment of arthritis. The most common being, ginger, willow bark extract, Chinese thunder god vine, cat's claw, stinging nettle and feverfew.

Though there is some evidence that extract of willow and ginger help to relieve pain, they do contain properties that are remarkably similar to non-steroidal anti-inflammatory compounds like ibuprofen and naproxen, FDA approved medications. The thing to bear in mind; is both the herbal and manufactured options can cause some inflammation in the intestines and stomach; they may also affect persons with heart conditions or hypertension.

Despite the fact that Chinese thunder god vine helps relieve inflammation and pain, constant use can weaken the bones and immune system.

Asthma

Most medications prescribed for this condition tend to trigger horrible side effects. Herbal remedies help cut down on the incidences of these side effects as lower dosages can be taken. Of course, always consult with the doctor before making any alterations to dosage.

Asthma is a Greek word, traditionally Greeks brewed anise seeds and fennel seeds to make a tea to help not only with asthma but other respiratory conditions. The tea was made by putting a heaped teaspoon of each seed in a pestle where they were cracked and then steeped in about a pint of boiled water for approximately fifteen minutes. It was then sipped warm. The effects were calming and reduced the spasms that typically come with an attack. A component alpha-Pinene helps to free you from bronchial secretions. Black or green tea also helps with asthma as they contain theophylline, a chemical that relaxes the muscles in the bronchial tubes.

Another effective remedy is licorice root. This is deemed a great detoxifier in Chinese medicine and can be used with other herbs to cut down on their side effects. Licorice has anti-diuretic properties and should not to be used by an individual with high blood pressure.

For the treatment of asthma, licorice root helps augment the effectiveness of cortisol which cuts down on the need to use lots of steroids. Another compound found in the licorice root, glycyrrhizin, allows an individual to take lower doses compared to taking the full dosage of prednisolone, a manufactured drug to treat asthma and lupus.

A natural anti-inflammatory, ginger, helps to lower the process of inflammation which typically occurs with asthma and allergies. Other compounds like silybin from milk thistle and curcumin from turmeric help as well.

If one wants to stimulate the adrenal glands to reduce inflammation by releasing corticosteroids, yerba mate is rather effective. It works to dilate the bronchial tubes and relax the airways.

Another well-known herb used in the treatment of asthma, cold and allergies is Ephedra. Misuse of this drug has received some bad press. Ephedra should be used cautiously as it can cause an increase in the level of the user's blood pressure and heart rate.

Certain Types of Depression

The most popular herbal treatment for depression is St. John's Wort. It has been the subject of many studies and has been shown to have a significant effect on relieving anxiety and relieving depression after a month of use. It rarely triggers any side effects. In extremely rare cases there may be instances in which the user may experience sensitivity to sunlight. The consumption of pickled herring, red wine, cheese and yeast should be avoided while taking St. John's Wort.

It is important to take care of one's nutritional needs. Without proper nutrition the brain cannot makes neurotransmitters. One must also have the right amounts of folate and Vitamin B6. Consumption of sunflower seeds, asparagus, citrus fruits, parsnips, spinach, beets and dark green leafy vegetables will provide the necessary amounts of each.

Pumpkin seeds also provide copious amounts of the amino acid tryptophan which helps with the synthesis of serotonin, a neurotransmitter. Serotonin causes a feeling of well-being.

Another option for depression is aromatherapy. Rosemary, geranium, mint, lavender, chamomile and angelica all help to lift the users' spirits. A massage with a combination of these oils does not hurt either.

Another herbal remedy ginkgo biloba helps the brain to produce certain neurotransmitters that can help alleviate depression.

Canker Sores and Cold Sores

Herbs that work well to alleviate the symptoms of canker sores include but are not limited to chamomile, Oregon grape root and Echinacea. A mouthwash can also be made from these herbs and used to speed up the healing process.

If licorice is used it is best to take it for a short period of time while the cold sore is present or to use it topically. A commercial version of licorice, known as deglycyrrhizinated licorice (DGL for short) works well at healing canker sores without raising blood pressure.

Cold sores have to be treated by herbs with antiviral properties. St. John's Wort and lemon balm can be applied to the areas as soon as the tingling that precedes the cold sore is noticed. It can be used several times per day as long as the sore is present. Oregon grape has some antiviral properties as well and the use of licorice keeps the virus from replicating.

Immune boosters like Echinacea can help to stave off the herpes virus. Echinacea helps protect the skin from succumbing to the attacks from viral and bacterial enzymes. When it is taken internally it is very effective.

Chamomile also helps to heal sores that occur in the mucous membranes and has some anti-microbial properties of its own.

Canker Sore Recipe

*¼ teaspoon licorice root (powdered)
*¾ cup water (lukewarm)
*The licorice root should be stirred into the lukewarm

water. It should then be used to wash the mouth for two to three minutes morning and evening until the sores are all healed.

Cold Sore Recipe

*1 tablespoon lemon balm (freeze dried or fresh)
*1 cup water (boiling)
*The boiling water should be poured over the lemon balm and allowed to steep for fifteen minutes. It can then be had as a tea and can be cold or hot. You can have as much as you want. A few cups a day will help with herpes. The dried lemon balm should not be used unless it was picked and dried by you and still has a strong smell.

Eczema

The babul tree bark is a potent form of treatment for eczema. It is to be boiled and then the fumes are used to stimulate the areas that are affected.

The seeds of the Butea tree are also effective. It is effective when mixed with lime water and applied to the affected areas.

Linseed oil can also be mixed with lime water and applied to the affected areas. It also helps with other skin ailments as well.

Oil can be extracted from the leaves of the Madhuca and then applied to the areas that are affected.

Dietary Treatments for Eczema

Outlined below are a few dietary practices that must be adhered to by eczema patients:

- Reduce the amount of salt in the diet.

- Avoid sour foods like curds and pickles.

- Something with a bitter taste is good like bitter drumstick or bitter gourd. The flowers from the neem tree are also good.

- Turmeric is a great soother for the skin. It can be used liberally when flavoring food. It can also be applied to the affected areas to provide relief.

Problems with Menstruation and Menopause

Cimicifuga Racemosa or Black Cohosh is a woodland perennial and a part of the buttercup family. The root can be boiled and drunk as tea and helps ease labor pains and menstrual cramps. Recent studies have also shown that is effective at minimizing the emotional issues like weepiness, mood swings and depression that come with menopause. It also helps ease hot flushes.

Important points to note are that black cohosh does not mitigate the hot flashes experienced during menopause. It can also be bought as a coloring or in tablet form.

At least one occasion has been cited of a female that has contracted autoimmune hepatitis from taking this herb.

Studies that have been done have not made any connection between liver toxicity and the use of black cohosh. Of course if you have problems with your liver it is best to be cautious and not use it.

Endemic to southwest China, dong quai is a plant extract. It is typically combined with other products to provide relief from the symptoms of menopause.

Evening primrose oil is known to help relieve pain in the breasts. Two prescription versions of this oil that used to be sold are Epogam and Efamast can help with symptoms of eczema and breast pain respectively. It can now be easily be bought without a prescription and goes under the name of borage oil as well. It is sold in varying potencies and strengths. One can simply look for the level of gamma linoleic acid (GLA) that is contained in the capsule. It is advised that you take at least two hundred and forty milligrams daily for two months then reduce the dosage. Some people that have used this have experienced nausea, headache and skin rashes.

A remedy made from extracts of pollen that also helps reduce the symptoms of menopause is Femal. It helps with hot flashes and also improved the users' general mood, reduced dizziness, mood swings, improved libido and tiredness.

Ginkgo Biloba otherwise known as the maidenhair tree is known to improve circulation and memory. It also enables more oxygen and glucose to go to the brain.

A root endemic to Peru, Maca has high levels of essential amino acids, minerals, vitamins and enzymes. It is purported to help boost libido and hormone production.

Sage in tablet form or as a tea helps with the hot flushes. The studies are still being done on this herb.

The very popular St. John's Wort helps relieve the symptoms of depression and anxiety as mentioned beforehand. It works just as well as the traditional medications and helps women that have problems with depression and anxiety as a result of menopause. It does not interact well with some medication so verify with your doctor before taking it.

Chapter 3: Herbal Remedies For Allergies

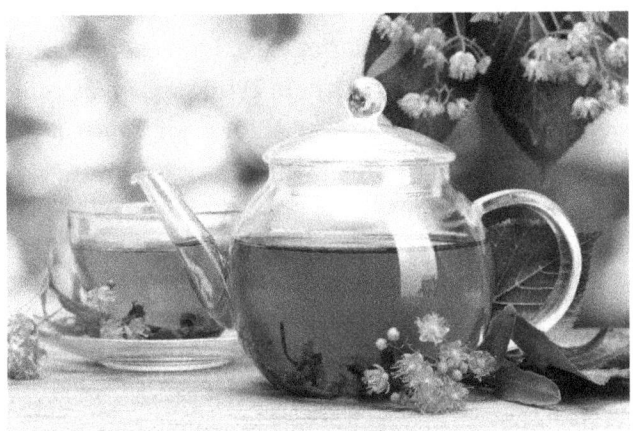

For persons that have issues with hay fever, nature can be the worst thing ever. Hay fever can be defined as the allergic reaction to pollen. The typical symptoms are a thin nasal discharge, sneezing, itchy, watery and inflamed eyes.

Though the allergies can be anywhere from agonizing to mildly uncomfortable there are a few herbal remedies that can offer some form of relief.

Herbal Remedies for Allergies

A natural antihistamine, Vitamin C helps to cut down on the level of nasal inflammation and drainage. Flavonoids that work well with this vitamin are hesperidin, quercetin and rutin. Certain foods like citrus fruits, broccoli, spinach, plums and berries have both.

Nettle is another remedy that helps cut down on the symptoms of hay fever. A tincture can be made from the leaves and used daily. It can also be found in tablet form or simply used as a tea. The nettle cuts down on the level of histamine that the body produces. If a tablet of three hundred milligrams is taken daily most people find relief for a few hours.

Butterbur is a weed found in Europe. This weed got its name from the fact that the leaves were used to wrap butter when refrigeration as we know it did not exist. Studies found it was just as effective as the active ingredient in Zyrtec known as cetirizine. It works well as an antihistamine and does not cause drowsiness. However, one has to be careful however as it can cause symptoms to worsen in some individuals.

Angelica also helps provide relief. It has properties that block the production of certain antibodies that are the result of an allergic response. A half teaspoon in a cup of water makes a great tea.

Licorice helps reduce the level of inflammation as it enhances the level of cortisol in the body. It has no known detrimental side effects.

Cayenne or Chili Pepper contains capsaicin. This ingredient helps prevent the excess secretion of fluids from the nasal cavity when a person is exposed to pollen or some other irritant.

The great thing in all of this is that allergies can be controlled. A lot of the traditional medications are just meant to treat the symptoms and not the underlying condition. With herbs one can get to the root of the problem and prevent the symptoms from even occurring.

There are a few things that one can do to help control exposure to allergens.

- A window fan is a big no-no as it can pull the pollen indoors.

- When driving, the windows should be kept closed. If necessary, the air conditioner can be utilized to help avoid exposure to allergens.

As much as possible, try to stay indoors when the pollen count is at its highest. This is usually from the middle of August until the first frost.

Chapter 4: Dealing With Digestive Problems

Battling Bouts of Nausea, Motion Sickness, Morning Sickness, Vomiting, Heartburn, Dyspepsia, Bloating, Belching, Flatulence or Diarrhea

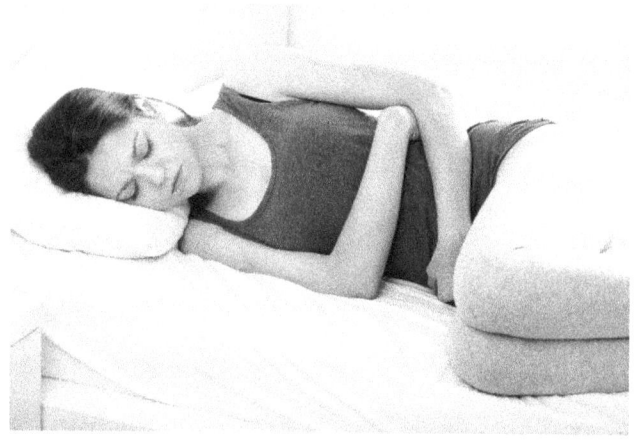

What Are Botanical Nervines?

Problems that occur in the digestive are often linked to tension, anxiety and stress. Herbs known as botanical nerviness are preferred as they work to not only boost the nervous systems but have a positive effect on the digestive system as well.

These nerviness work by reducing the response to stress which is the way in which the nervous system responds in an emergency situation by cutting off all bodily functions that are not required in survival mode so to speak. The herbs counteract all of this by calming the user down and settling the stomach.

The most important thing that has been constantly highlighted throughout this book is the important traits that herbal medicines or phytotherapy has, which a few of these plants have adaptogenic or biphasic effects. This simply means they have overlapping or complementary actions based on what is going on in the body.

With nerviness, some herbs can perform the double function of being stimulant nerviness (stimulating stagnant or lax tissues as it relates to the nervous system) or as relaxant nerviness (relaxing tissues that are contracted or constricted as it relates to the nervous system). Others work as form of nutrients for the nervous system. Outlined below are five nervines that aid in the process of digestion.

Peppermint

The benefits derived from peppermint are mostly from the aromatic phenols and oils that buildup in the trichomes. Essential oil of peppermint has been used for centuries as a digestive aid. Now there is the scientific backing to support the claims of how it works.

The delayed release capsules work best as it gets to go through the upper gastrointestinal tract right through to the lower intestine where it can dissolve and relax the muscles, reduce digestive spasms, relieve gas, reduce discomfort and pain as well as slowing down contraction in the gastrointestinal tract. Caution is to be exercised however as high doses can have adverse effects. Persons with kidney stones, GI reflux or hiatal hernia should seek medical advice before taking.

Peppermint can also be used topically. Add a few drops of peppermint oil to hot water, soak a towel in it and place it over the abdomen for approximately half an hour. This can be done up to three times per day and is a great treatment for distention or bloating.

Persons not affected by any digestive disorder can enjoy peppermint as a tea. There are no adverse effects from this. It is widely consumed and is a nice soothing end to dinner.

Chamomile

Chamomile works well to alleviate digestive symptoms. It can be used homeopathically, as a tisane or a tincture. It has long been used as a form of relief for chronic and acute gastric distress such as cramps or inflammation in the digestive organs as it has anti-inflammatory and anti-microbial properties.

The chemical compounds of chamomile are being isolated and studied. It is deemed safe except for persons that are allergic to plants in the onion, celery or sunflower families.

Lemon Balm Rosemary and Valerian

Typically combined, valerian, rosemary and lemon balm are three last nervines that will be highlighted. They aid with the relief of gassiness, digestive spasms, pain and queasiness. There is not a lot of scientific data on these herbs but they have been noted to be well tolerated.

Lemon balm is a member of the mint family and has also been used for years to relieve the symptoms of spasms, dyspepsia and gas. Rosemary has antispasmodic effects and has similar properties to lemon balm. They both have a compound known as rosmarinic acid. Valerian is best known for helping with nervous sleep disturbance and restlessness and is often combined with lemon balm or hops and used as a sedative. It has long been used to help with viral gastroenteritis, colic, nausea, flatulence, cramps and constipation.

Other Herbal Digestive Aids

Fennel

A form of Ayurvedic medicine, fennel seeds and leaves are known to help relieve constipation, relieve gassiness, heartburn and bloating. It is also thought to be able to help with improving appetite. Babies with colic are usually giving some tea made with fennel and some other herbs or as an emulsion of fennel seeds. Allergic reactions are rare.

Ginger Root

This root has been used for so long that it cannot even be said where exactly its use started. It has the ability to strengthen the stomach and reduce the effects of vomiting and nausea. The active compounds gingerals works as inhibitors of prostaglandins (pro-inflammatory chemicals). Formulations including ginger have been used to relieve queasiness at sea and on land and it has even been tried in space. Women in their first trimester of pregnancy use it as well to help with morning sickness.

Ginger is antiemetic, antiulcer, anti-motion sickness, anti-secretary, gastric secretory, antioxidant, antimicrobial and anti-nauseate. It can be had as a tea or juice, encapsulated or dried powder, decoctions or fresh gingerroot.

Digestive Bitters

Bitters can be a tincture, distillation or tincture of aromatic roots, fruits, barks and herbs that have a number of medicinal qualities. The overall purpose is to improve digestion. Quite a number of mixtures exist that have been successfully passed down from one generation to the next. The most popular to date is Swedish bitters which had its beginnings in sixteenth century Europe and was used to treat a number of conditions including stomach cramps.

Angostura bitters which is thought by most to be for cocktails was originally made to help with stomach ailments. Add a few drops of mineral water and it can aid with digestion and work well as an alternative to fruit juices, sugary sodas and alcoholic beverages. It has a rather refreshing taste.

Digestive Herbs - Not Only for Taste

The herbs highlighted are but a few of the many herbs that can aid with digestive problems. These herbs can typically be found in your local grocery or health food store, at an herbalist or naturopath or even in your own backyard garden. Keep in mind that persons will react differently to treatments and that there are a lot of other options to alleviating digestive problems.

The following point cannot be made enough- consult with a doctor or qualified herbalist before starting any form of herbal treatment.

Herbal Preparations – A Few Terms

What exactly is the difference between a tincture, decoction, tisane and infusion? The differences are outlined below.

Tincture is an extract that is made by placing plant material or herbs in a jar with a form of alcohol like ethanol and allowing it to steep for a few weeks before it is strained. At times glycerin or vinegar is used in its place.

Decoction is made by boiling mashed or ground up plant materials in water before straining it.

Tisane is a brewed herbal tea that is made from any plant but Camellia Sinesis (the real tea plant).

Infusion is like a decoction or tisane but tends to be more potent. The plant materials are usually soaked in boiling water or oil for a while.

Chapter 5: General Problems

Ear, Nose and Throat

There are a few conditions that can affect us from time to time. They are not life threatening and can range from your standard earache to sore throat or runny nose. Herbal treatments are available that can help alleviate the symptoms.

Natural Remedy for Ear Aches

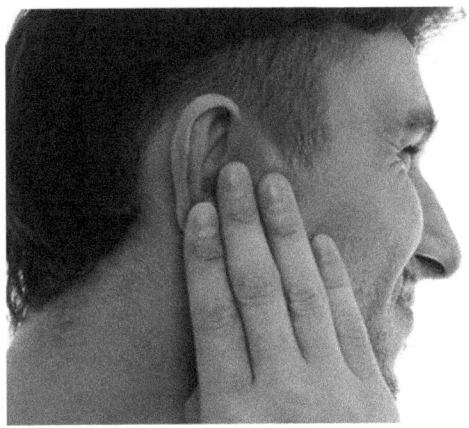

Pain in the ear usually indicates an ear infection. There are few steps that can be taken to alleviate this condition.

A quick check with the local pharmacy will reveal a lot of options. There is, for example, a garlic oil or Vitamin E oil capsule. They can simply be warmed in hot water and used in the ear.

Chamomile is also a great option to help relieve the infection. It should be warmed and wrapped in a cloth and then placed against the affected ear. It can be done with a cold compress as well where an ice bag is placed against the ear for about fifteen minutes.

Ginger is not for stomach aches alone, it works well for earaches. A fresh piece of ginger should be grated and mixed with sesame oil. Equal amounts of the juice should then be dropped in each ear. After that is done a cotton ball is to be used to plug each ear. This will keep foreign matter out.

Natural Remedy for Runny Nose

Another common problem though annoying is a runny nose. The dripping is not only a nuisance but embarrassing at best. If it is not dealt with from in its early stages it can develop into something worse like sinus problems, a cough or even an earache. It can even lead to all three.

One home remedy to deal with a runny nose is to dissolve a tablespoon of salt in eight ounces of warm water. This solution can then be used to wash the nostrils. A dropper can be used to dispense the solution. Slowly inhale the solution and keep doing it until some relief is felt.

The herb, thyme is typically used for cooking, it can also work effectively against a runny nose. One or two tablespoons of thyme should be finely crushed and should be as close to powder form as possible when you are done. Once crushed, the powder can be inhaled.

Turmeric is another great option. Soak ground turmeric is to be soaked in linseed oil and apply heat until it starts to smolder. The smoke is to be inhaled to relieve the runny nose.

Herbal Remedies for Sore Throat

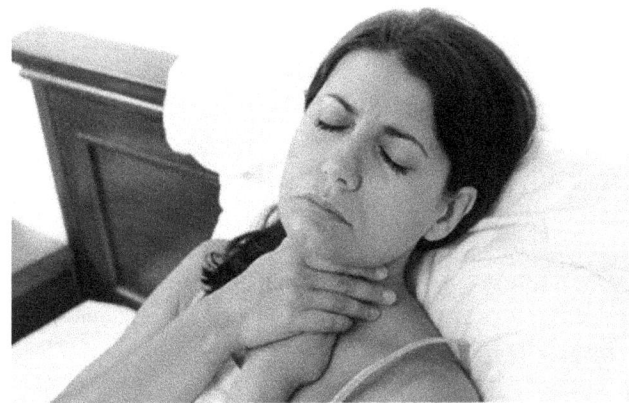

A sore throat cannot be ignored as it is usually an indicator of another problem. Relief must be found quickly for this condition. A few natural options are outlined below that help reduce inflammation and ease pain.

Goldenseal or Echinacea boost the immune system and relieve the symptoms of sore throat as a result of flu or cold.

Garlic helps to fend off bacteria and viruses that can trigger illnesses. It can simply be added to the diet.

Blackberry or Raspberry Leaves can be used to make a solution that can be used for gargling to relieve the discomfort.

Cayenne Pepper can be used in solutions that you gargle with to help stop the pain of a sore throat.

Getting Professional Help

Though herbal remedies are deemed effective against these general health problems the symptoms are not to be ignored. The herbal methods are best used in the initial stages or as preventative methods. It is best to have a doctor examine you to ensure that everything is okay.

If you use natural remedies and the conditions listed below are still prevalent a doctor should be seen immediately.

- The condition is ongoing (for several days or more).
- When it is difficult to breathe or swallow as the result of a sore throat.
- When blood is in phlegm or saliva.
- When a fever is present.

Herbal Remedies - The Benefits

One of the primary advantages of making use of herbs is that they are safer than the manufactured options. It is also much less expensive as you will probably have most products in the house already. The great thing is that more natural ingredients are being used with many traditional medications.

CHAPTER 6: WHY I LOVE FLAXSEED OIL

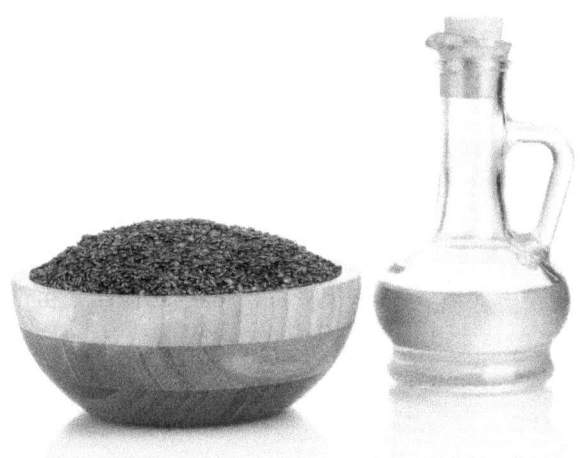

The Health Benefits of Flaxseed Oil - An Herb Remedy

Flaxseed is a well know source of fiber. Studies have indicated that it does have health benefits as it contains omega 3 fatty acids that are very successful at treating lupus and cardiac ailments.

Flaxseed also helps lower cholesterol, keep blood pressure stable and prevent certain heart diseases. Persons that have had heart attacks in the past can always take some flaxseed oil as a preventive measure. Flaxseed oil works well for heart disease, acne, high blood pressure, arthritis, menstrual cramps, depression and breast cancer. Taking it on a regular basis can alleviate or prevent these conditions from occurring.

If the problem is constipation, flaxseed oil can help as it enables free bowel movement. If the intestinal tract is inflamed it will help in the repair process. It is also effective at preventing the occurrence if gallstones or dissolving ones that are present.

This oil can also help with certain skin issues. These include sunburn, rosacea, eczema and acne. It prevents the cracking and breaking of the skin and keeps it moisturized.

The debilitating effects of Alzheimer's disease can also be alleviated with the use of flaxseed oil.

It can be bought in liquid form or as a capsule. This is why some persons prefer to add it to their meal instead of vegetable oil. It can be used in any baked product like bread or in beverages. No more than three grams should be consumed.

The best way to keep it is to refrigerate it or store it in a cool dark place. It is made from freshly pressed seeds and is usually bottled in dark containers and the processing is done at low temperatures without light, heat and oxygen.

MEET THE AUTHOR

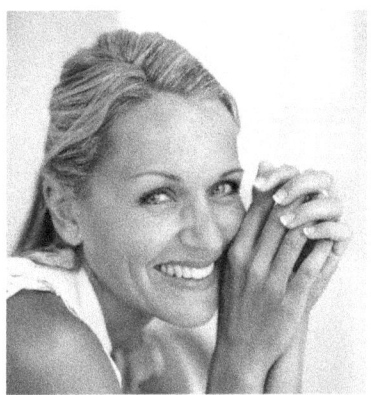

Angela Curtis has spent most of her adult life learning about herbs and the effects that they can have on certain illnesses that plague mankind. From the wealth of knowledge she has garnered "Herbal Remedies Explained" was born. She outlines the various properties of the most common herbs and how they work to heal the body. A few recipes (if you want to term them as such) are outlined as well for some simple yet effective home remedies.

Angela puts everything together in a few chapters but she could go on and on as these herbs do work on more than one illness. The ones highlighted are the most common like asthma and eczema. Even issues with the ear, nose and throat are covered.

One thing that Angela does not deviate from is the fact that no matter what you may have diagnosed by yourself, a medical professional should be consulted before any herb or combination of herbs is taken. This is vital as the wrong amounts can be taken which might trigger some adverse effects.

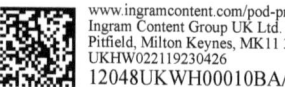
www.ingramcontent.com/pod-product-compliance
Ingram Content Group UK Ltd.
Pitfield, Milton Keynes, MK11 3LW, UK
UKHW022119230426
12048UKWH00010BA/606